AROMATHERAPY

For Beginners

Guide To Essential Oils, Blends, And Techniques For Health, Wellness, And Relaxation - Harness The Healing Power Of Nature To Enhance Your Mind, Body, And Spirit

ROBERT LUGO

CHAPTER 1 4

Introduction To Aromatherapy 4

CHAPTER 2 10

Basics Of Aromatherapy 10

CHAPTER 3 14

Aromatherapy Tools And Equipment 14

CHAPTER 4 19

Popular Essential Oils And Their Properties 19

CHAPTER 5 22

Aromatherapy Techniques And Applications 22

CHAPTER 6 25

Aromatherapy For Specific Conditions 25

CHAPTER 7 29

Blending Essential Oils 29

CHAPTER 8 33

Incorporating Aromatherapy Into Daily Life 33

CHAPTER 9 37

Aromatherapy And Holistic Health 37

CHAPTER 10 46

Aromatherapy For Special Populations 46

CHAPTER 11 49

Exploring Advanced Aromatherapy 49

CHAPTER 12 52

Aromatherapy Case Studies And Success Stories 52

Conclusion 55

CHAPTER 1
Introduction To Aromatherapy

Aromatherapy, often regarded as a holistic healing practice, utilizes essential oils extracted from plants to promote physical, emotional, and psychological well-being. This therapeutic approach harnesses the aromatic compounds found in these oils, which are believed to possess various healing properties. Through inhalation, topical application, and sometimes ingestion under expert guidance, aromatherapy seeks to enhance the body's natural ability to heal and restore balance. It is deeply rooted in ancient practices and continues to evolve as a complementary therapy in modern healthcare.

What is Aromatherapy?

At its core, aromatherapy is the art and science of using aromatic plant extracts, specifically essential oils, to improve one's overall health and well-being.

These oils, derived from flowers, leaves, stems, roots, and other parts of plants, are concentrated essences that capture the plant's beneficial properties. Aromatherapists carefully select and blend these oils to create synergistic effects that address specific health concerns, ranging from stress relief and relaxation to pain management and skin care. The therapeutic use of aromatherapy extends beyond its pleasant scents; it involves understanding the chemical composition and therapeutic actions of each oil for targeted therapeutic benefits.

History and Origins of Aromatherapy

The origins of aromatherapy can be traced back thousands of years to ancient civilizations such as Egypt, Greece, China, and India. These cultures recognized the healing potential of aromatic plants and used them in rituals, medicine, and perfumery. The Egyptian practice of embalming, for instance, involved the use of aromatic substances like myrrh and frankincense. In ancient Greece, Hippocrates, the "Father of

Medicine," advocated the use of aromatic baths and scented massages for their therapeutic effects. Similarly, traditional Chinese medicine and Ayurveda integrated aromatic herbs and oils into their healing practices. The modern concept of aromatherapy emerged in the early 20th century, pioneered by figures like René-Maurice Gattefossé and Marguerite Maury, who explored the therapeutic benefits of essential oils and laid the foundation for its contemporary application in healthcare.

Aromatherapy's Advantages and Applications

Aromatherapy offers a wide range of benefits and applications across physical, emotional, and mental health domains. Some of the key benefits include stress reduction and relaxation, improved sleep quality, pain relief, immune support, enhanced mood and emotional balance, cognitive enhancement, skincare and haircare benefits, respiratory support, and digestive aid. The diverse uses of aromatherapy encompass massage therapy, inhalation techniques (such as diffusers and steam inhalation), topical applications (like aromatherapy massage oils and skincare products), aromatic baths, compresses, and more. Each essential oil carries unique properties that contribute to its specific therapeutic benefits, allowing for customized blends tailored to individual needs and preferences.

Safety Guidelines and Precautions

While aromatherapy is generally considered safe when used appropriately, it is essential to observe safety guidelines and precautions to avoid potential risks or adverse reactions. Some key considerations include:

1.   Dilution: Essential oils are highly concentrated and potent, requiring dilution with carrier oils or other mediums before direct skin application to prevent skin irritation or sensitization.

2.   Patch Testing: Before using a new essential oil or blend, conduct a patch test on a small area

of the skin to check for any allergic reactions or sensitivity.

3.   Pregnancy and Medical Conditions: Certain essential oils may not be suitable for pregnant women, infants, young children, or individuals with specific medical conditions.

Consultation with a qualified aromatherapist or healthcare provider is advisable in such cases.

4.   Quality and Purity: Choose high-quality, pure essential oils from reputable sources to ensure efficacy and safety.

Avoid synthetic fragrances or adulterated oils that may lack therapeutic benefits and could pose health risks.

5.   Storage and Handling: Store essential oils in dark, airtight containers away from heat, light, and moisture to preserve their potency and integrity. Follow proper handling procedures to prevent accidental spills or exposure.

Adhering to these guidelines ensures the safe and effective use of aromatherapy, maximizing its therapeutic benefits while minimizing potential risks. With knowledge, caution, and respect for the potency of essential oils, individuals can experience the transformative power of aromatherapy in enhancing their well-being naturally.

CHAPTER 2
Basics Of Aromatherapy

Aromatherapy, often referred to as essential oil therapy, is a holistic healing approach that harnesses the aromatic compounds of plants to promote physical, emotional, and mental well-being. At its core, aromatherapy relies on the therapeutic properties of essential oils, which are volatile substances extracted from various plant parts such as leaves, flowers, stems, and roots. These oils contain concentrated natural compounds that have been used for centuries in traditional medicine and healing practices.

Essential Oils: Definitions and Extraction Methods

Essential oils are highly concentrated plant extracts that capture the essence, aroma, and beneficial properties of plants. They are obtained through various extraction methods such as steam distillation, cold pressing, solvent extraction, and effleurage.

Steam distillation is the most common method and involves passing steam through plant material to extract the essential oil, which is then condensed and collected. Cold pressing is used for citrus fruits, where the oils are extracted by pressing the peels. Solvent extraction involves using solvents like hexane to extract oils from delicate plant parts. Enfleurage is a traditional method where flowers are placed on a fatty substance to absorb their oils.

Carrier Oils and Their Importance

Carrier oils play a crucial role in aromatherapy as they dilute essential oils and help deliver them safely to the skin. They are often derived from seeds, nuts, or kernels and have their therapeutic properties. Jojoba, almond, coconut, and olive oils are examples of common carrier oils.

These oils not only dilute the potent essential oils but also provide nourishment and hydration to the skin. Choosing the right carrier oil depends on factors like skin type, the desired therapeutic effect, and personal preferences.

Comprehending Aromatherapy Blends

Aromatherapy blends are combinations of essential oils and carrier oils designed to create specific therapeutic effects. Blending essential oils requires an understanding of each oil's properties, such as its aroma, therapeutic benefits, safety considerations, and compatibility with other oils. Blends can be tailored for various purposes, such as relaxation, stress relief, immune support, pain management, and skincare. The art of blending involves experimenting with different oils and proportions to achieve desired results while ensuring safety and efficacy.

Quality Assessment and Purchasing Tips

Ensuring the quality of essential oils is paramount in aromatherapy to reap their full therapeutic benefits. Quality assessment involves considering factors such as purity, potency, source, extraction methods, organic certification, and third-party testing for contaminants. It's essential to purchase oils from reputable suppliers who provide detailed information about their products, including botanical names, country of origin, extraction methods, and safety guidelines. Price should not be the sole determinant of quality, as high-quality oils may be more expensive due to their purity and potency. Conducting research, reading customer reviews, and consulting with aromatherapy experts can help in making informed purchasing decisions.

CHAPTER 3
Aromatherapy Tools And Equipment

Aromatherapy Tools and Equipment play a crucial role in harnessing the therapeutic benefits of essential oils for beginners and enthusiasts alike. Understanding these tools and how to use them effectively is key to maximizing the potential of aromatherapy in daily life.

Diffusers: Types and Usage Diffusers are essential devices that disperse essential oils into the air, creating a fragrant and therapeutic atmosphere. There are several types of diffusers available, each with its unique features and benefits:

1.   Ultrasonic Diffusers: These diffusers use ultrasonic vibrations to break down essential oils into micro-particles, which are then dispersed into the air as a fine mist. They are popular for their quiet operation and ability to maintain the therapeutic properties of oils.

2.   Nebulizing Diffusers: Nebulizers do not require water or heat to disperse oils. Instead, they use pressurized air to create a fine mist of pure essential oil particles. This type of diffuser is preferred for its strong and direct aroma delivery.

3.   Evaporative Diffusers: These diffusers use a fan to blow air through a pad or filter containing essential oils. The air then carries the aroma into the surrounding space. They are simple to use and suitable for smaller areas.

4.   Heat Diffusers: Heat diffusers use heat to evaporate essential oils and release their aroma into the air. While they are easy to use, they may alter the chemical composition of oils and reduce their therapeutic benefits.

Understanding the usage of each diffuser type is essential for beginners to choose the right one based on their preferences and needs.

Inhalers and Roll-Ons for Aromatherapy Inhalers and roll-ons are portable and convenient ways to experience aromatherapy benefits on the go.

1.   Aromatherapy Inhalers: These are small tubes containing a cotton wick soaked in essential oils. Users inhale the aroma directly from the inhaler, which can help with stress relief, respiratory support, and mood enhancement.

2.   Aromatherapy Roll-Ons: Roll-ons are diluted essential oil blends that are applied directly to the skin. They are commonly used for topical applications, such as for relaxation, pain relief, or skincare purposes.

Both inhalers and roll-ons are user-friendly options for beginners to incorporate aromatherapy into their daily routines.

Aromatherapy Candles and Incense Aromatherapy candles and incense are popular choices for creating a calming and aromatic ambiance at home or in therapeutic settings.

1.   Aromatherapy Candles: These candles are made with essential oils infused into the wax. When the candle burns, it releases the aroma of

the oils into the air, providing a soothing and aromatic experience.

They are often used for relaxation, stress relief, and mood enhancement.

2.   Aromatherapy Incense: Incense sticks or cones infused with essential oils can be burned to release fragrant smoke. They are used in meditation practices, relaxation rituals, and to purify the air while imparting therapeutic benefits.

Choosing high-quality aromatherapy candles and incense is important to ensure the purity and effectiveness of the essential oils used.

Storage and Preservation of Essential Oils Proper storage and preservation of essential oils are essential to maintain their potency and effectiveness over time.

1.   Dark Glass Bottles: Essential oils should be stored in dark glass bottles to protect them from light, which can degrade their quality. Amber or

cobalt blue bottles are commonly used for this purpose.

2.   Cool and Dry Environment: Essential oils should be stored in a cool, dry place away from direct sunlight and heat sources. Excessive heat and light can cause oils to deteriorate and lose their therapeutic properties.

3.   Airtight Seal: Ensure that the bottles containing essential oils are tightly sealed to prevent air exposure, which can lead to oxidation and degradation of the oils.

4.   Labeling and Date: Properly label each bottle with the name of the oil and the date of purchase or creation. This helps track the shelf life of oils and ensures that they are used within their recommended timeframe.

CHAPTER 4
Popular Essential Oils And Their Properties

Popular essential oils are key components in aromatherapy, offering a wide range of therapeutic benefits. Lavender oil, derived from Lavandula angustifolia, is renowned for its calming and relaxing effects. Its gentle aroma has been used for centuries to promote relaxation, alleviate stress and anxiety, and improve sleep quality. Lavender oil's soothing properties make it a popular choice for aromatherapy enthusiasts seeking emotional balance and tranquility in their daily lives.

Peppermint oil, extracted from Mentha piperita, is prized for its invigorating and refreshing properties. The menthol content in peppermint oil provides a cooling sensation that can help relieve headaches, boost energy levels, and enhance mental alertness. Its stimulating aroma is often used to combat fatigue, improve concentration, and promote a sense of vitality.

Peppermint oil is a versatile addition to aromatherapy blends, offering both physical and mental benefits to users.

Tea tree oil, sourced from Melaleuca alternifolia, is renowned for its antimicrobial and healing benefits. This potent essential oil is widely recognized for its ability to combat bacteria, fungi, and viruses, making it a popular choice for addressing various skin concerns such as acne, fungal infections, and minor cuts or wounds.

Tea tree oil's purifying properties also extend to its use in household cleaning products and natural remedies for respiratory congestion.

Eucalyptus oil, derived from Eucalyptus globulus or Eucalyptus radiata, offers respiratory support and decongestant properties. Its camphoraceous scent is commonly used to alleviate symptoms of colds, coughs, and sinus congestion. Eucalyptus oil is often added to steam inhalations or diffused to promote clearer breathing and relieve respiratory discomfort.

Additionally, its analgesic properties can provide relief from muscle aches and pains when used in topical applications or massage blends.

Each of these popular essential oils brings unique benefits to aromatherapy practices, offering users a holistic approach to health and wellness. Incorporating these oils into daily routines can enhance mood, support physical well-being, and create a harmonious environment conducive to relaxation and rejuvenation.

CHAPTER 5
Aromatherapy Techniques And Applications

Aromatherapy Techniques and Applications encompass a wide array of methods and practices that utilize essential oils for therapeutic purposes. Understanding these techniques is crucial for beginners to effectively harness the benefits of aromatherapy.

Inhalation Methods form a cornerstone of aromatherapy practices. Steam Inhalation involves adding essential oils to hot water and inhaling the steam, allowing the aromatic molecules to enter the respiratory system and exert their therapeutic effects. Diffusion, another popular method, uses devices like diffusers to disperse essential oil particles into the air, creating a soothing and aromatic ambiance.

Topical Application involves applying diluted essential oils directly to the skin.

Massage is a common technique where oils are blended with carrier oils and used in gentle, therapeutic massages to promote relaxation, relieve muscle tension, and improve circulation. Compresses involve soaking a cloth in a diluted essential oil solution and applying it to specific areas of the body for localized relief. Bathing with essential oils added to bathwater is another way to enjoy their benefits through absorption and inhalation simultaneously.

Room Sprays and Environmental Fragrancing are methods used to enhance the atmosphere and mood of a space. Room sprays are simple mixtures of essential oils and water, sprayed into the air to freshen the room and create a pleasant scent. Environmental fragrancing involves using diffusers or sachets to continuously release essential oil aromas into the environment, promoting relaxation, focus, or other desired effects.

Aromatherapy for Emotional Well-being is a significant aspect of its application.

Certain essential oils are known for their mood-enhancing properties, such as lavender for relaxation, citrus oils for uplifting moods, and frankincense for grounding and centering. Aroma therapists often create customized blends to address specific emotional needs, offering support for stress relief, anxiety management, mood elevation, and overall emotional balance.

By exploring and understanding these Aromatherapy Techniques and Applications, beginners can embark on a journey of holistic wellness and self-care, harnessing the power of nature's essences to enhance physical, mental, and emotional well-being.

CHAPTER 6
Aromatherapy For Specific Conditions

Aromatherapy offers a diverse range of benefits for specific conditions, making it a popular choice for individuals seeking natural remedies. When it comes to stress and anxiety management, aromatherapy harnesses the power of essential oils to promote relaxation and calmness.

Oils like lavender, chamomile, and bergamot are known for their soothing properties, helping to reduce stress levels and alleviate anxiety symptoms. Inhalation of these oils through diffusers or steam inhalation can have a calming effect on the mind and body, making aromatherapy a valuable tool in stress management techniques.

Sleep disorders, particularly insomnia, can significantly impact one's quality of life. Aromatherapy offers a holistic approach to sleep support, with essential oils such as lavender, cedarwood, and valerian root known for their sleep-inducing properties. These oils can be used in bedtime rituals, such as adding a few drops to a bath, diffusing them in the bedroom, or applying diluted versions to pulse points.

Aromatherapy promotes relaxation, reduces sleep disturbances, and helps create a conducive environment for restful sleep, making it a valuable addition to sleep hygiene practices.

Headaches and migraines are common ailments that can be debilitating for many individuals. Aromatherapy provides a natural alternative for headache relief, with oils like peppermint, eucalyptus, and rosemary known for their analgesic and anti-inflammatory properties.

Inhalation of these oils or topical application through massage or compresses can help alleviate headache symptoms, reduce pain intensity, and promote overall well-being. Aromatherapy's gentle yet effective approach to headache relief makes it a preferred choice for those seeking non-pharmacological remedies.

Skincare is another area where aromatherapy shines, offering a range of benefits for various skin conditions. Essential oils like tea tree, lavender, and rosehip are renowned for their skincare properties, including anti-inflammatory, antibacterial, and moisturizing effects.

Incorporating these oils into skincare routines through serums, creams, or facial steams can help address acne, eczema, dryness, and other skin concerns.

Aromatherapy promotes healthy skin by nourishing and rejuvenating the skin barrier, making it a valuable tool in natural skincare practices.

Aromatherapy for specific conditions encompasses a holistic approach to wellness, harnessing the therapeutic benefits of essential oils for stress and anxiety management, sleep support, headache relief, and skin care.

By understanding the properties and uses of various essential oils, individuals can integrate aromatherapy into their daily lives to enhance overall well-being and promote a healthier lifestyle.

CHAPTER 7
Blending Essential Oils

Blending essential oils is a fundamental aspect of aromatherapy that combines the art and science of aromatics to create customized blends for various purposes. Understanding the basic principles of blending is crucial for beginners venturing into the world of aromatherapy.

The process involves combining different essential oils to achieve specific therapeutic effects, taking into account factors such as scent profiles, therapeutic properties, and safety considerations.

One of the primary principles of blending essential oils is synergy, which refers to the combined effect of oils working harmoniously together to enhance their therapeutic benefits. This principle emphasizes the notion that the combined action of multiple oils can be more potent and effective than individual oils used alone.

Synergy also involves balancing the aroma of the blend to create a pleasing and balanced scent profile.

Another key principle is dilution, which involves blending essential oils with carrier oils or other diluents to reduce the concentration of the pure essential oil. This is essential for ensuring safety, as some essential oils can be highly potent and may cause skin irritation or other adverse reactions if used undiluted. Understanding the appropriate dilution ratios based on age, health status, and intended use is vital for safe and effective blending.

Creating personalized aromatherapy blends is a creative process that allows individuals to tailor their blends to address specific health concerns, emotional states, or personal preferences.

This involves considering factors such as the desired therapeutic effects, preferred aromas, and individual sensitivities or allergies.

By experimenting with different combinations of essential oils, individuals can discover unique blends that resonate with their needs and preferences.

Aromatherapy recipes provide structured guidelines for blending essential oils to achieve specific therapeutic goals. These recipes often include detailed instructions on the types and quantities of essential oils to use, as well as the recommended dilution ratios for different applications such as massage oils, diffuser blends, or bath salts. Beginners can benefit from exploring a variety of aromatherapy recipes to gain insight into the art of blending and the diverse range of therapeutic possibilities.

Blending for different methods of application involves adapting blends to suit various delivery systems, such as topical application, inhalation, or diffusion. Each method of application offers distinct benefits and considerations, influencing the choice of essential oils and their concentrations in the blend. For example, blends intended for topical use may focus on skin-nourishing oils with soothing properties, while inhalation blends may prioritize oils that support respiratory health and emotional well-being.

Blending essential oils in aromatherapy is a multifaceted process that combines scientific knowledge with creative exploration.

By understanding the basic principles of blending, creating personalized blends, exploring aromatherapy recipes, and adapting blends for different methods of application, beginners can embark on a rewarding journey of holistic wellness and self-care through aromatherapy.

CHAPTER 8
Incorporating Aromatherapy Into Daily Life

Incorporating aromatherapy into daily life can significantly enhance well-being and promote a sense of relaxation and balance. Aromatherapy is a versatile practice that can be integrated into various aspects of daily routines, from household chores to personal care and work environments. Let's delve into how aromatherapy can be effectively used in different settings:

Aromatherapy at Home: Cleaning, Laundry, and Air Freshening

Aromatherapy can transform mundane household tasks into therapeutic experiences. Using essential oils in cleaning solutions adds a pleasant fragrance while also providing antimicrobial properties.

For instance, tea tree oil is renowned for its antibacterial and antifungal properties, making it an excellent addition to surface cleaners.

Lavender oil not only leaves a calming scent in the laundry but also has relaxing effects, promoting a peaceful ambiance in the home. In air freshening, diffusing citrus oils like lemon or orange can uplift the mood and create an invigorating atmosphere.

Aromatherapy in the Workplace

Incorporating aromatherapy into the workplace can boost productivity, reduce stress, and improve overall well-being. Diffusing essential oils such as peppermint or eucalyptus can enhance focus and mental clarity, ideal for office environments. Citrus oils like bergamot or grapefruit can create a refreshing and energizing atmosphere, helping employees stay motivated throughout the day. Aromatherapy can also be used during breaks or meetings to promote relaxation and reduce tension.

Aromatherapy for Travel and Stress Relief

Traveling can be stressful, but aromatherapy offers a portable and effective solution for relaxation on the go.

Using a personal inhaler or diffuser with calming oils like chamomile or lavender can help reduce travel-related anxiety and promote restful sleep during long journeys. Peppermint oil is excellent for combating travel fatigue and boosting energy levels. Additionally, aromatherapy can be incorporated into travel essentials such as neck pillows or hand sanitizers for added comfort and wellness benefits.

Aromatherapy in Personal Care Products

Many personal care products can benefit from the inclusion of aromatherapy ingredients. Incorporating essential oils into skincare products like lotions or serums can offer both aromatic and therapeutic properties. For example, adding rosemary oil to hair care products can promote scalp health and stimulate hair growth.

Aromatherapy can also enhance the sensory experience of baths and showers by using aromatic bath salts or shower steamers infused with relaxing oils like ylang-ylang or cedarwood.

By integrating aromatherapy into daily life through these various avenues, individuals can experience the holistic benefits of essential oils in promoting physical, mental, and emotional well-being. Whether at home, at work, during travel, or in personal care routines, aromatherapy offers a natural and enjoyable way to enhance daily experiences and nurture a healthier lifestyle.

CHAPTER 9
Aromatherapy And Holistic Health

Aromatherapy and Holistic Health

Aromatherapy, as a holistic approach to health and well-being, delves into the intricate connections between scent, emotions, and physical wellness. The foundation of aromatherapy lies in the use of essential oils extracted from plants, each possessing unique therapeutic properties.

These oils are carefully selected and blended to create synergistic effects that promote balance within the body and mind. The holistic philosophy of aromatherapy encompasses not just the physical benefits of essential oils but also their impact on the mental, emotional, and spiritual aspects of wellness.

The holistic perspective in aromatherapy views individuals as interconnected beings, where imbalances in one aspect can affect the whole.

Essential oils are utilized to address these imbalances, aiming for a harmonious equilibrium that supports overall health. This approach considers factors such as lifestyle, diet, stress levels, and emotional state in crafting personalized aromatherapy solutions. By integrating aromatherapy into a holistic health framework, practitioners and enthusiasts alike can tap into the profound healing potential of nature's aromatic treasures.

Integrating Aromatherapy with Massage Therapy

The integration of aromatherapy with massage therapy creates a powerful synergy that enhances the therapeutic benefits of both modalities. Massage therapy, known for its ability to relieve muscle tension, improve circulation, and promote relaxation, becomes even more effective when combined with the targeted use of essential oils. Aromatherapy adds an extra dimension to the massage experience, amplifying its healing effects on both the body and mind.

Essential oils used in conjunction with massage therapy are selected based on their specific properties and desired outcomes. For instance, lavender oil, renowned for its calming and soothing properties, is often incorporated into massages aimed at reducing stress and inducing relaxation. Peppermint oil, with its invigorating and cooling effects, may be used in massages focusing on pain relief and revitalization.

The application of aromatherapy during massage can be tailored to individual preferences and needs. Whether through diffusing essential oils in the massage room, adding them to massage oils or lotions, or using them in hot compresses, the aromatic elements heighten the sensory experience and deepen the therapeutic impact of the massage session.

This integration of aromatherapy with massage therapy offers a holistic approach to well-being, addressing both physical tension and emotional balance.

The incorporation of aromatherapy into yoga and meditation practices enriches the mind-body connection, facilitating deeper states of relaxation, focus, and mindfulness. Essential oils, with their potent aromatic compounds, complement the transformative nature of yoga and meditation, creating an immersive sensory experience that enhances the practice.

During yoga sessions, aromatherapy can be introduced through diffusers, inhalers, or applied topically before or after practice. Oils such as frankincense, known for their grounding and spiritually uplifting properties, are favored choices for yoga sessions focused on introspection and connection. Citrus oils like orange or bergamot may be used to invigorate and energize during dynamic yoga practices.

In meditation, aromatherapy aids in creating a conducive environment for deepening concentration and relaxation. Lavender oil, renowned for its calming effects, promotes a sense of tranquility and mental clarity, making it a popular choice for meditation spaces. Sandalwood and cedarwood oils, with their earthy and grounding aromas, can deepen the meditative experience, fostering a sense of inner peace and stability.

The synergy between aromatherapy and yoga or meditation extends beyond the physical practice, nurturing a holistic approach to well-being that encompasses body, mind, and spirit.

By incorporating aromatic elements into these practices, individuals can enhance their ability to enter states of mindfulness, presence, and inner balance.

Aromatherapy and Ayurveda

Aromatherapy and Ayurveda, ancient healing systems rooted in natural principles, share a common goal of restoring balance and promoting health through holistic means. Ayurveda, often referred to as the "science of life," recognizes the interconnectedness of body, mind, and spirit in maintaining well-being. Aromatherapy, with its focus on the therapeutic properties of essential oils, aligns seamlessly with the principles of Ayurveda, offering additional tools for healing and rejuvenation.

In Ayurveda, essential oils are categorized according to their doshic qualities, aligning with the three doshas—Vata, Pitta, and Kapha—that represent different elemental energies within the body. This classification guides the selection of oils based on an individual's unique constitution and any imbalances present. For example, warming oils like ginger or cinnamon may be used to balance Vata imbalances characterized by dryness and cold, while cooling oils like rose or jasmine help pacify excess Pitta related to heat and inflammation.

The integration of aromatherapy into Ayurvedic practices expands the therapeutic repertoire, offering personalized solutions for addressing specific health concerns.

Essential oils are used in various Ayurvedic therapies such as Abhyanga (Ayurvedic oil massage), Shirodhara (oil pouring therapy), and aromatic steam treatments. These applications harness the aromatic potency of oils to nurture physical vitality, emotional balance, and mental clarity in alignment with Ayurvedic principles.

By synergizing aromatherapy with Ayurveda, practitioners gain a comprehensive approach to holistic healing that honors individual constitution, elemental balance, and the interconnectedness of body, mind, and spirit.

This integration embodies the timeless wisdom of ancient healing traditions enriched by the therapeutic art of aromatherapy.

Aromatherapy to Promote Emotional and Mental Calm

Aromatherapy's profound impact on mental and emotional well-being stems from its ability to influence mood, cognition, and stress response through scent.

Essential oils, with their complex aromatic profiles, interact with the limbic system in the brain, which governs emotions, memories, and behaviors. This neurological connection forms the basis for using aromatherapy as a therapeutic tool for achieving mental and emotional balance.

Certain essential oils are renowned for their mood-enhancing properties. For instance, lavender oil is celebrated for its calming and anxiety-reducing effects, making it a valuable ally in promoting relaxation and stress relief. Citrus oils such as lemon or orange uplift mood and promote a sense of vitality and positivity. Rosemary and peppermint oils are known for their invigorating and clarifying effects, enhancing mental focus and cognitive function.

In addition to individual oils, aromatherapy blends are crafted to target specific emotional states or concerns. Blending lavender with bergamot and ylang-ylang, for example, creates a synergistic blend that promotes relaxation, uplifts mood, and fosters emotional balance.

These customized blends can be diffused, applied topically, or incorporated into self-care rituals to support mental well-being.

Aromatherapy's role in emotional balance extends to holistic approaches for managing stress, anxiety, depression, and sleep disorders. Integrating aromatherapy into daily routines, mindfulness practices, and therapeutic interventions offers a natural and complementary avenue for enhancing mental resilience, emotional harmony, and overall quality of life. This holistic perspective acknowledges the interconnectedness of mental, emotional, and physical aspects of well-being, emphasizing proactive self-care and natural healing modalities.

CHAPTER 10
Aromatherapy For Special Populations

Aromatherapy for special populations encompasses a range of considerations and tailored approaches to maximize the benefits of essential oils while addressing the unique needs and sensitivities of different groups. Aromatherapy for children and babies involves careful selection and dilution of essential oils to ensure safety and effectiveness.

Children's skin is more delicate and prone to irritation, so gentle oils like lavender, chamomile, and mandarin are commonly recommended. These oils can help promote relaxation, improve sleep quality, and alleviate common childhood issues like colic or anxiety.

Elderly and seniors can also benefit greatly from aromatherapy, but considerations such as medication interactions and skin sensitivity become more critical.

Gentle oils like lavender, rosemary, and frankincense are often used to support relaxation, mental clarity, and joint health. Aromatherapy can complement elderly care by providing a non-invasive way to address common concerns like sleep disturbances, mood swings, and cognitive function.

Aromatherapy for pets is gaining popularity as a natural way to support their well-being. However, it's essential to use pet-safe oils and avoid those that can be toxic to animals. Oils like lavender, chamomile, and peppermint, when used in moderation and with guidance from a veterinarian, can help calm anxious pets, repel insects, and support overall health. Dilution and proper application methods are crucial to ensure safety and effectiveness.

Pregnancy and postpartum care present unique considerations for aromatherapy due to hormonal changes and the need for gentle, supportive approaches. Many essential oils are contraindicated during pregnancy, especially in the first trimester, so caution and expert guidance are essential. Oils like lavender, chamomile, and ylang-ylang can be used in diluted forms to promote relaxation, relieve nausea, and support emotional well-being during pregnancy and the postpartum period.

Each of these special populations requires a tailored approach to aromatherapy, considering factors like age, health conditions, and safety considerations. Consulting with a qualified aromatherapist or healthcare professional is advisable to ensure the safe and effective use of essential oils for these groups.

CHAPTER 11
Exploring Advanced Aromatherapy

In delving into advanced aromatherapy, one must first grasp the intricate chemistry underlying essential oils. Aromatherapy Chemistry: Understanding Constituents delves into the molecular composition of essential oils, elucidating the roles of terpenes, phenols, aldehydes, ketones, esters, and more. Understanding these constituents not only aids in comprehending the therapeutic properties of oils but also guides advanced blending techniques.

Advanced Blending Techniques elevate aromatherapy from mere scent to profound therapeutic efficacy. This section delves into the art of blending oils for specific purposes, such as stress relief, immune support, pain management, and emotional balance. Techniques like layering, dilution ratios, and synergy creation are explored in depth, empowering practitioners to craft potent and personalized blends.

Aromatherapy's integration with Traditional Medicine showcases its evolution from alternative practice to respected complementary therapy.

By examining the historical uses of aromatics in cultures worldwide, this section highlights the synergy between traditional healing modalities and modern aromatherapy.

Case studies and research findings validate the efficacy of aromatherapy alongside conventional treatments, fostering collaboration and holistic wellness approaches.

Looking towards the future, Future Trends and Innovations in Aromatherapy forecast the exciting advancements shaping this field. From novel delivery systems like inhalers and patches to bioengineering scents for targeted therapeutic outcomes, the landscape of aromatherapy is expanding exponentially. Integration with digital platforms for personalized aromatherapy experiences and sustainability initiatives in sourcing and production also mark key trends driving the industry forward.

As practitioners delve into advanced aromatherapy concepts, they unlock new dimensions of healing and wellness, harnessing the power of nature's aromatic treasures for holistic health and vitality.

CHAPTER 12
Aromatherapy Case Studies And Success Stories

In exploring the realm of aromatherapy, one of the most compelling aspects lies in the wealth of case studies and success stories that illuminate its practical efficacy and transformative potential. These narratives not only provide a glimpse into the diverse applications of aromatherapy but also serve as testimonies to its profound impact on individuals' well-being across various contexts.

Real-life applications of aromatherapy span a wide spectrum, from personal wellness routines to clinical interventions. Testimonials and experiences shared by individuals who have integrated aromatherapy into their lives offer invaluable insights into its effectiveness in addressing physical, emotional, and mental health challenges. These firsthand accounts often highlight the nuanced ways in which different essential oils and blends can be tailored to meet specific needs, fostering a deeper understanding of aromatherapy's versatility and adaptability.

Case studies play a pivotal role in substantiating the therapeutic value of aromatherapy through systematic observation and analysis.

By documenting the outcomes of aroma therapeutic interventions in controlled settings or real-world scenarios, these studies contribute to the growing body of empirical evidence supporting its efficacy. From alleviating symptoms of stress and anxiety to enhancing sleep quality and promoting relaxation, case studies provide tangible evidence of aromatherapy's potential as a complementary wellness approach.

Tips for achieving long-term success with aromatherapy encompass practical strategies for optimizing its benefits over time. This includes guidance on selecting high-quality essential oils, understanding proper dilution and application methods, and establishing consistent routines for integration into daily life.

Emphasizing the importance of personalized approaches and ongoing self-care practices, these tips empower individuals to harness the full potential of aromatherapy as a holistic wellness tool.

By delving into aromatherapy case studies, real-life applications, testimonials, and long-term success tips, individuals can gain a comprehensive understanding of its multifaceted benefits and transformative possibilities. Whether embarking on a journey of self-discovery or seeking to enhance professional practice, the insights gleaned from these perspectives serve as invaluable resources for harnessing the power of aromatherapy in promoting health, harmony, and vitality.

Conclusion

As we conclude our journey into the world of aromatherapy, it's essential to reflect on the wealth of knowledge we've explored.

Aromatherapy is more than just the use of essential oils; it is a holistic practice with deep historical roots and numerous benefits for both body and mind. By understanding the history and origins of aromatherapy, we've gained insight into its long-standing significance and the science behind its therapeutic effects.

We've delved into the basics of aromatherapy, learning about the importance of essential oils and carrier oils, the methods of extracting these precious essences, and how to create effective and safe blends. With the right knowledge, selecting quality oils and using the proper tools and equipment becomes an easy and rewarding task, allowing you to maximize the benefits of your aromatherapy practice.

The properties of popular essential oils like lavender, peppermint, tea tree, and eucalyptus have been highlighted, showing their versatile applications for relaxation, invigoration, healing, and respiratory support.

These oils, when used with appropriate techniques and applications such as inhalation, topical application, and room fragrancing, can significantly enhance your well-being.

Aromatherapy is particularly powerful in addressing specific conditions such as stress, anxiety, insomnia, headaches, and skin issues. Personalized blends tailored to your unique needs can provide targeted relief and support, enhancing your quality of life.

Incorporating aromatherapy into daily routines, whether at home, work, or while traveling, offers practical ways to maintain a sense of balance and peace in our hectic lives.

Integrating aromatherapy with other holistic practices like massage therapy, yoga, and meditation can further amplify its benefits.

This synergy promotes not only physical relaxation but also mental and emotional balance.

Whether it's for children, the elderly, pets, or pregnant women, aromatherapy can be adapted to suit various special populations, making it an inclusive and versatile wellness tool.

For those looking to advance their knowledge, exploring the chemistry of essential oils, mastering advanced blending techniques, and staying informed about future trends in aromatherapy opens up new possibilities for innovation and deeper understanding.

Real-life case studies and success stories demonstrate the transformative power of aromatherapy, offering inspiration and practical tips for achieving long-term success in your practice.

As you continue your aromatherapy journey, remember that the key to effective practice lies in continuous learning, experimentation, and mindful application. Embrace the sensory delights and therapeutic benefits of aromatherapy, making it a cherished part of your daily life and overall wellness routine.

www.ingramcontent.com/pod-product-compliance
Lightning Source LLC
Chambersburg PA
CBHW051702250726
48653CB00007B/2803